The Green 'JUICE' detox diet Book.

The AMAZING

3-day detox diet.

Author: Oliver Michaels

THE GREEN JUICE DETOX DIET.

Thank you for your incredible support

Oliver Michaels.

ISBN-13:
978-1482585995

ISBN-10:
1482585995

Inner **BODY** healing, detoxifies **Your** liver, Helps to **rebuild your blood cells**, **Boosts** **your** immune system, Stabilizes **blood** sugar, Reduces FOOD CRAVINGS, Improves skin PROBLEMS and overall complexion, **Builds** **stronger** hair & **Stronger** nails, Removes toxins **from your body**, Improves your digestion, Improves mental clarity, Increases **your** ENERGY **and** Promotes weight **loss, burns** out Stubborn **fat**, **Lowers** your **Cholesterol**, **STOPS** **Premature** ageing, prevents development of cancer, Studies show can **also** help to **remove** cancer cells.

Dedication

This book is dedicated to my mother Jean Redshaw Emmett who died in August 2008 after a long battle with breast cancer.

I will never forget your amazing strength you showed us all, I love you and miss you every single day...x

TABLE OF CONTENTS

INTRODUCTION

THE GREEN JUICE DETOX DIET

The Green Juice detox diet is an amazing 1–3 day guide to detox your body with 'easy to make' recipes feeding your body with nutrients, anti-oxidants phytonutrients, vitamins and minerals you need. In this book you will learn about your body, the function of your organs and what diet is most beneficial for you. Learn about toxins, parabens, food additives and the affect they have on your body and your everyday life.

Find out what foods are beneficial to your body and why.

The amazing 3-day detox-diet plan is a healthy new start that is educational, entertaining, inspirational, and an overall dramatic boost to a healthy lifestyle...

This book will show you how to detoxify safely, feel good and achieve quick weight loss results, also by changing a few habits in your diet you can easily maintain your new you.

REVIEW...

"AMAZING, an enlightenment and education of our amazing bodies, and how to care for them... thank you Oliver Michaels..."

ABOUT THE AUTHOR.

Oliver Michaels was born in Newcastle England, 3 years ago he moved to North America where he now lives with his family.

Oliver has no MEDICAL degrees or NUTRITIONAL training what so ever...!

However, for the past 25 years he has suffered personally from wrong nutritional and medical diagnosis. He has endured 25 years of suffering with food intolerances, stomach cramps, digestion pains, acid indigestion, reflux and skin flares.

This has resulted in years and sometimes intrusive medical testing and medication.

Oliver has been diagnosed with IBS, suspected duodenal ulcer, lactose intolerance and suffered the effects of rosacea. He has had barium meals, ultra sound scans, CAT scans and recently 2010 had surgery for acute hydrophrenosis of the right kidney.

In August 2008 Oliver sadly lost his mother after she lost her long fight with cancer. It was after the loss of his mother he was driven to publishing his own experiences and findings in his book to what he describes as, *"the most amazing nutritional healthy plan and fast healing diet for your whole body".*

Oliver has an insatiable appetite for learning, researching and self-improvement. This book is a result of Oliver's 25 years of researching, suffering, misdiagnosis, dieting and his own research for a way to rid him of his severe stomach pains, digestion issues and gain overall health, fitness and wellness.

Oliver gives you over 30 healthy green juice recipes, all you will ever need. You also get his essential formula for creating your very own amazing juice recipes.

Oliver takes you on his personal quest for a healthy, pain free diet solution and offers you a simple easy argument as to why you should add a Green Juice Drink to your daily diet.

He also gives you the nutritional benefits and values of every fruit, vegetable and herb including the individual healing affects these have on your body… All this and so much more!

Today Oliver suffers little to no stomach or digestion discomfort, minimal stomach pains or bloating, he has great skin tone, hair and body tone and it's all from his discipline to follow The Green Juice detox diet.

A PERSONAL MESSAGE FROM THE AUTHOR.

Thank you for reading my book, I want to share this amazing diet with you, I sincerely hope you enjoy and achieve the amazing body healing benefits of juicing…

One to three juices NOT a SMOOTHIE a JUICE', every day, using green vegetables such as Celery, kale, cucumber, or spinach, has an amazing effect on your organ health, strengthens your immune system, promotes fat melting healthy weight loss… and so much more.

"So why NOT a Smoothie I hear you say?"…

Don't get me wrong Smoothie's are great and they are healthy, however they don't give you the same fast acting health benefits of Juicing.

Juicing is the only way of fully breaking down the fibres and then feed the live nutrients, vitamins, phytonutrient's and minerals directly into your liver, then directly into your blood stream.

Juicing provides you an amazing healthy and healing effect on your whole body, also improving, soothing and aiding your digestive system.

You will eat a wider variety of greens than you ever have before but now with total ease…

Before you start this amazing life changing diet…. let me just ask you one question…. Can you remember the last time you had a plate of celery, spinach leaves, parsley, kale ginger root or Swiss chard? …..

I do…

I juiced some this morning…..!

Enjoy your new diet …it's amazing.

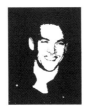

Oliver Michaels

Please feel free to email me should you have any questions or queries regarding your new juice diet. olivermichaels.author@hotmail.com

Thank you for your incredible support, I hope you like it.

AWAKEN YOUR BODY'S OWN HEALING MECHANISMS.

Throughout my researching into Juicing, detoxing and dieting, I discovered that detoxing is world renown as a completely natural healing therapy that has been used for thousands of years in helping to aide, treat, and even cure many common ailments.

Your body is already capable of instigating its own perfect detox healing if you allow it the opportunity. Detoxing and dieting your body with the right balance of vitamins, minerals and phytonutrient's, is that opportunity.

While modern medicines so often attempt to alleviate your outer symptoms of a health condition, I quickly learned that juicing aids your healing from the inside out.

The Juicing detox-diet gets to the actual source of your condition, helping to regenerate your inner body. It is truly amazing, juicing burns out stored fat and inferior cells and helps you to build new healthier cells and tissues.

The daily intake of toxins into the body are rejected through your bodies amazing defence process and filtered by your liver and kidneys. Toxins are then expelled around your body as fatty deposits.

The Juicing detox dieting helps rid your body of the stored toxins (fatty deposits) and makes for healthier weight loss and an increase in energy levels.

Detox diets are methods of dieting that are normally used to shed extra pounds, but the major health benefits are often over shadowed and sometimes taken for granted.

The additional benefits of detoxing and consuming the juice diet are to help improve your health but also include massive healing benefits supporting a healthy glow to your skin, strengthening you hair- nails, helps to give you a flatter stomach, the feeling of being less bloated and giving you more energy.

Throughout this book you will discover the massive health benefits that the right detox diet can create which affects us on all levels of our lives and enhances us in so many different ways.

You will also be given the best guidance, including amazing low cost 'easy to make' recipes, a guide to understanding your body. Also you get a simple food, nutrients and benefits guide for fruits vegetables and herbs used in the diet.

Guidance on the essentials for making healthier food, information on how to make your whole detoxing and juice diet experience beneficial, long term and more enjoyable.

You can also follow the *'easy to make'* recipe plans and there's help to design and make your own 2 minute recipes using the ingredient list described in chapter 6.

DETOX-DIET the right way and keep away from the methods and diets that can cause you to yo-yo diet, feel permanently fatigued and can potentially disrupt your body's balance.

If you are planning or researching a detox, then *this book is a MUST read...!* You can review and follow the course time and time again, with simple to follow recipes for your own healthy and successful Juicing detox-juicing diet plan.

CHAPTER 1

JUICING DETOX DIETING, IS THIS REALLY HEALTHY FOR US?

This is something I spent a lot of time looking into, I didn't want to accept the answer I believed. I *wanted* to actually look at what happens when you drink a Smoothie, a Juice or eat raw food. How does our body interpret these diets and what is the best healthy diet for us.

The truth is some detox plans can be very healthy, but in some other cases detox–dieting may not be safe!

As you have read your body auto detoxes for you on a daily basis. This is part of our amazing body's auto defence, regeneration, repair and healing process.

So when you complete the *'Juice'* detox then the *'Juice'* diet you are boosting, accelerating, and aiding your body's natural process. The objective of the detox and juice diet is to rid your body of the stored toxins while still having the full respect for your body and all its functions.

A juicing detox and diet with fruits and vegetables gives you lots of anti-oxidants in each meal, with nutrients phytonutrients and vitamins that help to assist your body, especially your organs to cleanse and detoxify with ease and far less fatigue.

The Juicing detox-diet when done properly is the most amazing health benefit you can give your body…but you need to know why you're detoxifying and how to do it properly. You need to learn how to detox the right way.

The Juicing detox-diet plan (sometimes referred to as Juicing) is a healthy and safe dieting and occasional detox method but only if done properly. Juicing provides contrast with those of you who are of good health.

The juicing Detox should only be completed, and here's one of the key health benefit, for one to three days maximum, with a frequency of no sooner than once a month and no more…

The next stage is to then maintain the diet to heal your body from the inside, lose stubborn weight by burning out fat gained in difficult to lose areas, and massively improve your overall health.

WHAT ARE THE HEALTH BENEFITS AND HOW DOES JUICING WORK?
So the main health benefit of a fresh juicing detox diet is that your body can absorb MORE of the vitamins and minerals than if you were to eat the fruits and vegetables whole…!

Many of the nutrients are TRAPPED in the fibre and by juicing the fruits and vegetables you break down the fibre and release the vital nutrients directly into your body.

Some books are claiming you should detox for 8 days, 10 days and even 21 days or more, well this can be dangerous (unless carried out with professional guidance and advice) and if done frequently may result in starving your body of protein and throwing your body out of its natural balance.

By starving your body of protein you can do more harm than good to your most vital organ, your liver. You are thereby outweighing the overall affects and health benefits of your detox.

WHAT TOXINS DOES MY BODY ABSORB?

Well just through absorption the eliminating toxins you are exposed to everyday include, chemicals and parabens, our skin absorbs and you breathe toxins in to your body, you also eat foods containing parabens, artificial colours and preservatives every day, these are all foreign to your body.

Parabens are a class of chemical and are an effective preservative compound used for their bacterial and fungicidal properties that you will find in shampoos, moisturizer, shaving gels, topical/parenteral pharmaceuticals, makeup, spray tanning solutions, tooth paste but are also heavily used as food additives too.

Their efficiency as a food preservative combined with their low cost, the long history of use, and the inefficiency of natural alternatives such as grapefruit seed extract, is why parabens are so commonplace and still used extensively today.

They are becoming increasingly controversial however because in July 2002 a Dr. S. Oishi of The Department of Toxicology at Tokyo Metropolitan research lab had found parabens in breast cancer tumours. Reports have also shown that parabens display the ability to mimic estrogen (a hormone known to be linked to the development of breast cancer).

However no direct links between parabens and cancer have been fully established yet..!

Aspartame is an artificial, non-saccharide sweetener used as a sugar substitute in some foods and beverages. It was first sold under the brand name Nutra Sweet since 2009 it also has been sold under the brand name Amino Sweet.

The health concerns and safety of aspartame has been the subject of several political and medical controversies and internet hoaxes. Since its initial approval for use in food products by the U.S Food and Drug Administration (FDA).

It was in 1974 and by regulatory agencies in more than 100 countries a 2007 medical review on the subject concluded "the weight of existing scientific evidence indicates that aspartame is safe at current levels of consumption as a non-nutritive sweetener".

However, because its breakdown products include phenylalanine, aspartame must be avoided by people with the genetic condition phenylketonuria or PKU (an inherited disorder of metabolism that can cause intellectual and developmental disabilities (IDDs) if not treated).

The low calorie sweetener aspartame has been in use for 37 years and they say it is the most thoroughly tested ingredient in our food supply. It is made from two amino acids, the building blocks of protein that occur widely in the food we eat every day.

They are found in eggs, meat, cheese, fish, cereals, fruit and milk. Aspartame has been approved by the Food and Drug Administration (FDA), by experts of the United Nations Food and Agriculture Organization and the World Health Organization, and by regulatory agencies in more than 100 countries. Hmmm…!!

Refined Sugar, why is it Toxic to my Body?

It's hard to believe but **refined sugars** are **lethal** when ingested by humans because they provide what nutritionists describe as "empty" or "naked" calories. Refined Sugar lacks any natural minerals that are found in the natural sugar beet or sugar cane.

In 1957, Dr William Coda Martin tried to answer the question: When is a food a food and when is it a poison?

His working definition of "poison" was: Medically "Any substance applied to the body, ingested or developed within the body, which causes or may cause disease".

"Physically: Any substance which inhibits the activity of a catalyst which is a minor substance, chemical or enzyme that activates a reaction".

Even if you don't eat chocolate, sweets or candy, the amount of refined sugar you may be consuming would no doubt shock you. Over approximately 2/3 TWO-THIRDS of the refined sugars consumed around the world are refined sugars added to manufactured food products. In other words, sugar is hidden in many of the things we buy every day.

Did you know that a tablespoon of ketchup contains a full teaspoon of sugar? Also breads, soups, cereals, cured meats, salad dressings, spaghetti sauce, beans, crackers, mayonnaise, peanut butter, pickles, frozen pizza, canned products like fruits and vegetables, soups, tomato juice, and a host of other products all contain refined sugar. We haven't even taken into account the obvious sugary products like sweets, candies, cakes, ice cream, cookies, doughnuts, and fizzy pop drinks like Pepsi and coke.

Even if you are careful about reading the food and product labels, it's difficult to tell just how much refined sugar you're actually consuming. Sugar comes in many forms and guises, several of which might be contained in a single product.

Look out for terms like sucrose, fructose, glucose, and maltose.

In addition, refined sugar drains and leaches the body of precious vitamins and minerals through the demand its digestion, detoxification and elimination makes upon your entire body and system.

So essential is the balance to your body that your body has many ways to provide against the sudden shock of a heavy intake of sugar.

Minerals such as sodium (from salt), potassium and magnesium (from vegetables), and calcium (from your bones) are mobilized and used in chemical transmutation, neutral acids are produced which attempt to return the acid-alkaline balance factor of the blood to a more normal state.

Your body works extremely hard during a sudden intake of sugar which results in the initial energy surge then the major energy crash afterwards.

Sugar taken every day produces a continuously over acid condition, and more and more minerals are required from deep within your body in the attempt to rectify the imbalance.

Finally, in order to protect your blood, so much calcium is taken from your bones and teeth that this causes decay and then your bodies general weakening begins.

Excess sugar eventually affects every organ in your body. Initially, it is stored in the liver in the form of glucose (glycogen).

Since the liver's capacity to rid your body of the refined sugars is limited, a daily intake of this (above the required amount of natural sugar) soon makes your liver expand like a balloon.

When the liver is filled to its maximum capacity, the excess glycogen is returned to the blood in the form of fatty acids, massively increasing your cholesterol.

These fatty acids are taken to every part of the body and stored in your body's most inactive areas: your belly, arms, the buttocks, the breasts and the thighs in both men and women.

When these comparatively harmless places around your body are filled with fatty acids are then distributed among your active organs, such as the heart and kidneys.

These begin to slow down, finally their tissues degenerate and turn to fat. The whole body is affected by their reduced ability and abnormal blood pressure is created.

The parasympathetic nervous system is affected and organs governed by it such as the brain, become inactive or paralyzed.

The circulatory and lymphatic systems are then invaded, and the quality of the red corpuscles starts to change. An overabundance of white cells occurs and the creation of tissue becomes slower.

Our body's tolerance and immunising power becomes more limited, so we cannot respond properly to extreme attacks, whether that is cold, heat, mosquito bites or infections.

Your body has to prevent poisoning you every day, so all these toxins that are stored in fatty deposits around your body are sent there to prevent them from becoming toxic to your nervous system and your brain.

One of the benefits of a detox is to take these toxins from the fat tissue and get them out of the body through breathing, sweating and natural body waste.

In order for your body's ability to manage toxins affectively, you will need to have the foundation of a healthy diet which is free as much as possible of chemicals, pesticides, hormones, antibiotics, and very high in antioxidants, micronutrients, and phytochemicals.

You can achieve this by juicing, and further by introducing small changes into your everyday diet.

WATER

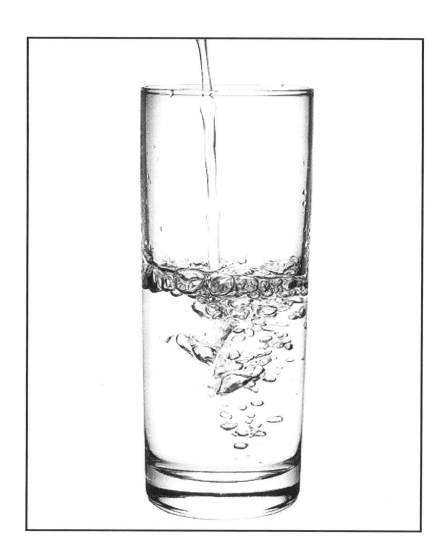

Statement: 80% of us are chronically dehydrated, we mistake our thirst for hunger and we tend to eat when our bodies are trying to tell us we are in fact thirsty and just need hydrated.

Yes most of us know this already…right…? But how many of us can honestly say we follow the guidelines for keeping us properly hydrated?

The health benefits of water.

Did you know that water is the body's main chemical compound and makes up a whopping 60% of your total body weight? All the systems in our body depend on water to maintain health.

Water flushes out toxins from our vital organs. Water carries nutrients to our cells and provides a moist environment for our ear, nose and throat tissue.

A lack of water can lead us to dehydration, and chronic health issues. Even without this juicing diet I urge you, if you want to vastly improve your health drink the recommended water intake daily.

How much water should I drink?

You lose water from your body through your breath, perspiration, urine and bowl movements. For your body to function properly we must replenish our water supply by consuming water and foods that contain water every day.

The institute of medicine recommends:

- MEN: 3.0 LITRES OR 10 CUPS A DAY.

- WOMEN: 2.2 LITRES OR 6-7 CUPS A DAY.

- PREGNANT WOMEN 2.4 LITRES OR 7 CUPS A DAY.

- BREAST FEEDING WOMEN: 3.0 LITRES A DAY OR 10 CUPS A DAY.

- EXERCISE: ADD AN EXTRA 2 TO 3 CUPS A DAY.

- ENVIRONMENT: HOT / HUMID WEATHER OR HEATED AIR TAKE IN EXTRA WATER.

- HIGHER ALTITUDES: INCREASED URINATION AND BREATHING, YOUR WATER INTAKE SHOULD BE INCREASED.

- SICKNESS: VOMITING, DIARRHOEA, BLADDER INFECTIONS AND URINARY TRACT STONES SHOULD ALSO INCREASE YOUR WATER INTAKE.

PLEASE NOTE:-

1 CUP OF WATER IS ON AVERAGE MEASURING 1/3 LITRE OR 333 ML. 1 TALL GLASS OF WATER IS ON AVERAGE MEASURING 425 ML.

Chapter 2

So why should we detox?

If you often feel tired, sluggish, have low energy or even low mood, feel bloated, or just suffer from general fatigue then your diet will be playing a major part in this.

Everyday life, the foods we eat and the environment you live in can all be hard on your body.

Junk food with synthetics, chemicals toxins, parabens, artificial colours, refined sugars, and flavours in our food, NON-organic foods laden with pesticides and hormones, to the cleaning products and environmental chemicals we breathe and absorb into our bodies EVERY DAY.

You are only equipped to deal with a certain degree of chemicals and toxin abuse in your body before this affects your overall health and wellbeing.

Well, it won't surprise you that your body could do with a break from the constant onslaught of your everyday life, diet and environmental chemicals you're subjected to.

Common side effects of the juicing detox-diet have resulted in increased bowl movements more frequently than usual daily. You may also feel slightly weak at the beginning of the detox, but hunger pains are very minimal providing you consume enough of the amazing juice daily.

People have reported that by the end of the 3 days they have an overall energy boost, loss of cravings and overall a healthier well-being. So initially during the detox people experience fatigue, but you must REMEMBER why you're doing the Juicing detox-diet in the first place…

Other symptoms may include nausea, irritability and headaches but these tend to show a greater need for a detox and tend to ease once the body has started eliminating some of the toxins. Most people also report radiant looking skin from the diet too.

Remember…the simple key to a healthy detox diet is to do a 1-3 days MAXIMUM detox, you don't want to starve your liver from protein and further affect your body's natural detoxing abilities and balance.

Your aim is to give your body the right foods so your organs can benefit from the richness in the vitamins, minerals and nutrients. Your body will then use these and their self-healing properties with improved efficiency all around your body. Making you feel healthier and more energised.

CHAPTER 3

DETOX DIET AND CLEANSE A BRIEF HISTORY.

Cleansing is a 5,000-year-old practice and not something new or one of these modern day fad diets. Detoxification is an alternative approach that proponents claim rids the body of "toxins", accumulated harmful substances that exert undesirable effects on an individual's health.

Detoxification usually includes one or more of, dieting, fasting, consuming exclusively, or avoiding specific foods (such as fats, carbohydrates, refined sugars) by eating fruits, vegetables, juices, herbs or water).

The premise of body detoxing and cleansing is based on the ancient Egyptian and Greek idea of autointoxication in which foods consumed can putrefy and produce toxins that harm the body.

Biochemistry to microbiology appeared to support the theory in the 19th century, but by the early twentieth century detoxification based approaches quickly fell out of favour.

Despite abandonment by mainstream medicine, the idea has persisted and become highly popular amongst healthy dieters, health gurus and alternative medicine practitioners.

In recent years, notions of body cleansing have undergone something of a revival along with many other alternative medical approaches.

However body cleansing is not yet supported by science, and with no medical benefits demonstrated it is not based on scientific claims. The toxins are usually undefined with no evidence for toxic accumulation in our bodies.

Now, based on the above information, only YOU can say if ridding your body of harmful modern day food additives and toxins like parabens and refined sugar can actually make you feel healthier and more energised.

There is however the other factors like the mass billion-dollar food industries impact and influence in the food market. This may be far too powerful for any scientific evidence to provide proof and endorse our beliefs.

CHAPTER 4

UNDERSTANDING YOUR INNER BODY.

Understanding your inner body's functions and needs, helps you to understand why and what you should be consuming in your diet every day, also I want to show you the direct affect your diet can have on your health and wellness.

YOUR LIVER:

This is the defence and the filter of the body. It is the largest organ inside your body. Did you know that an adult's liver is about the size of a football and it weighs close to three pounds?

Your Liver is located behind your ribs in the upper right-hand portion of your abdomen. It is dark reddish-brown and consists of two main lobes.

There are over 300 billion specialised cells in the liver that are all connected by a well-organized system of bile ducts and blood vessels called the biliary system.

SO HOW IMPORTANT IS YOUR LIVER?

It's your FIRST line of defence against toxins as it acts like a filter in preventing toxic substances (including drugs, alcohol) contained in foods and the environment from passing into your blood stream and especially into your brain and nervous system by converting them into harmless substances which then your kidneys can excrete through your urine. Your liver is such an important organ that we would only survive one or two days if it were to shut down.

If your liver fails, your body will fail too. Fortunately the liver can function even when up to 75% of it is diseased or removed. Your liver has the amazing ability to create new liver tissue and can regenerate itself using healthy liver cells that still exist.

So it's never too late to start looking after your liver and the rest of your body.

We all need to include anti-oxidants in our diet to keep us healthy. Vitamin - A, B3, B6, C, E, and beta-carotene as well as the amino acids L-Cysteine, L-Glutamine, glutathione and phospholipids are some of the real important ones.

SO WHAT DOES MY LIVER ACTUALLY DO?

Your liver does hundreds of vital things to make sure everything runs smoothly. Some of the most important functions of your liver include:

* Stores vitamins, sugar and iron to help give your body energy (cleansing the liver increases YOUR energy).

* Controls the production and removal of cholesterol (helps to eliminate high cholesterol levels).

* Clears your blood of waste products, drugs, and other poisonous substances.

* Makes clotting factors to stop excessive bleeding after a cut or an injury.

* Your liver produces immune factors and removes bacteria from the bloodstream to combat infection (improving your overall immunity health and wellness).

* Your liver also releases a substance called "bile" (this helps digest food and absorb important nutrients in your body).

The ratio of dietary protein to carbohydrate is a very important factor in determining the ability of the liver to function and detoxify certain substances successfully.

It deals with consumed food that contains fat when it enters your digestive tract before stimulating the secretion of cholecystokinin (CCK).

In response to CCK, your gallbladder, which can store about 50 millilitres of bile, then releases its contents into the duodenum.

The bile that is originally produced in your liver then emulsifies fats in partly digested food. Bile becomes more concentrated during storage in the gallbladder this increases its potency and intensifies its effect on fats.

Please remember if you have any health concerns or medical questions you <u>must</u> check with your family doctor before detox dieting or cleansing, especially if you suffer from diabetes or other dietary controlled ailments.

CHAPTER 5

ARE YOU READY TO CLEANSE YOUR BODY?

In the Amazing Juicing detox-diet plan we show you that detoxing is not all about deprivation and starvation - in fact it is quite the opposite.

Detoxing actually involves a total indulgence of your body's needs, consuming a healthy amount of vitamins, minerals, and phytonutrients, looking after yourself, and giving yourself the gift of a better body and a clearer mind.

BEFORE YOU START THE GREEN JUICE DETOX DIET.

FIRST, KNOW YOUR BODY AND KNOW YOUR LIMITS!!
Only you can decide if your body is ready for this. The diet follows a strict regime this only allows you to consume the juice drink and no solids may be eaten during the detox.

Note that I recommend your detox cleanse to be undertaken for no more than 3 days, this is to prevent any protein starving of your liver. This will be sufficient to provide your body with the boost of nutrients, anti-oxidants vitamins and minerals you need.

Also before starting the detox diet you need to stock up on some ingredients and apparatus that you will need.

Remember where possible buy organic farmed produce where you can, visit your local farmers market and ask about the produce you are buying, otherwise you're just putting chemicals and pesticides back into your body.

SELECTED FRUIT,

Apples, pears, peaches, pineapple (note high in sugar), lemons, limes, (note high in acids) tomatoes, blackberries, strawberries, grapes, oranges, watermelon.

SELECTED VEGETABLES,

Cucumber, kale (or lettuce), carrot, celery, radish, beetroot, spinach,

Cayenne Pepper, (this is a must and can be used in so many recipes)

Flax seed, Wheat grass, Ginger root, Purified or filtered water

1+ LITRE CHUGGABLE JUICE BOTTLES

A Sharp knife

Cutting board

Herbal laxative tea

Uniodized sea salt

1-teaspoon measure

The following are optional but give you more variety to your juicing detox-diet plan.

Cayenne Pepper said to be one of the most powerful herbs in the world.

Green tea, Peppermint tea, Colon cleanse, Liver cleanse

'Which' Power Juicer Guide.

So you need to buy a new juicer?... then follow this simple guide, I will give you the 5 features your need from your juicer. I then review the three best juicers at three different price points for you to choose from.

SO LET'S GET STARTED...

I'm not going to try to baffle you with the differing types of juicers, centrifugal juicers, masticating and twin gears this is a quick juicer review so you can buy a great machine and start juicing ...

5 MAJOR FEATURES YOU **NEED** FROM YOUR JUICER.

1.   The feeding tube diameter should be a min (3 inches) diameter, (most juicers are now) big enough for the whole fruits and vegetables to be fed down the tube without having to be sliced. When you start juicing you want to juice the whole vegetable or fruit without cutting if you can.

2.   The motor on the juicer should be no smaller than 800 watts to give you any longevity of your juicer and enable the juicing of whole fruits and vegetables without putting additional strain on the motor.

A variable speed motor is huge bonus. Heat and friction caused during the juicing process can kill some of the 'LIVE' nutrients…a similar process to pasteurisation in the food industry killing a lot of the nutrients thereby defeating the whole point of juicing in the first place.

3.   Cleaning the juicer is a frequent and can be an arduous task, make sure your new juice is easy to dismantle and easy to clean, look for this as a high ranking benefit or feature of your juicer, you will thank me later…

One useful tip…put a bag inside the pulp container saves on cleaning this container every time and allows for non-messy quick easy disposal). Also if you have compost bin then dispose of the pulp through your compost bin. Also buying a 'dish washer parts safe' model is a big bonus).

4.   Look at features like, stainless steel mesh filter, Be sure to get one with a steel cutting blade and a sleeve that isn't made of aluminum because it can react with the acids in fruit. A silent motor, spare juicing rotor blade and large pulp bin.

5.   Consider the height of the juice extraction port. It should be high enough to fit your tall glass underneath. This will save you transferring your juice drink from a short glass to a tall glass every time you juice.

My 3 personal juicer recommendations

"I've personally tried all three. They are at three different price points that will fit every budget"

The Hamilton Beach Big Mouth Juice Extractor

Cost price between $59.00 – $65.00

Available on Amazon.com.

Product Features

- *Yields up to 24% more apple juice than a leading competitor.*

- *You can fit the whole foods in the extra wide mouth for less pre-cutting, and comes with a pushing tool for easy juicing.*

- *With an extra-large pulp bin lets you juice longer without extra clean up.*

- *Easy to assemble and store. Comes with instructions booklet and cleaning brush.*

- *Powerful 800-watt motor for ease of use. Dishwasher safe parts.*

My Review

I have juiced large carrots, pears, apples, ginger roots, celery, kale, broccoli, spinach, and mango. For the most part the pulp that comes out is dry.

The metal mesh is really difficult to clean though. It does come with a brush that was affective. The rest of the juicer plastic is dishwasher safe. As per my advice the ease of cleaning is important.

My advice for this model is to hand clean it immediately after use. The only other thing I can really say is the height of the juice feeder is low so you can't fill your tall glass directly.

The feeding tube is large and easy to feed whole fruit and veggies down. Overall and for the money this is a very good juicer. Well-done Hamilton Beach.

My rating 3 * out of 5 *****

2. Jack Lalanne PJP Power Juicer Pro Stainless-Steel Electric Juicer
Cost price approx. $140.00

Available on Amazon.com.

Product Features.

- Extra-large round chute; stainless-steel blade and mesh filter

- Whisper-quiet 3,600 RPM motor; includes new patented extraction technology

- Large-capacity pulp collector; non-drip spout; dishwasher-safe parts

- Measures approximately 18 by 12 by 17 inches; comes with a limited lifetime motor warranty

Product Description.

Jack Lalanne has redesigned his best-selling juicer with a really smart looking new and sleek stainless steel finish and some really good new features, such as a non-drip spout and stainless steel mesh filter.

The Power Juicer Pro delivers a powerful 3,600-RPM of juicing.

My Review Jack Lalanne has redesigned of his best-selling juicer here, it has a new, sleek stainless steel finish and some great new features. Has a Non-drip spout and stainless steel mesh filter.

A powerful 3,600-RPM high performance motor with special extraction technology it is truly whisper quiet operation too. Also this has a lifetime warranty on the motor.

Lalanne claims it provides up to 30% more juice than other juicers, I did feel I was getting more juice but I am unsure of the percentage.

The unique non-drip spout and dishwasher-safe parts made it very easy to clean up.

I was very impressed with this juicer and found it so much fun to use, looks great in the kitchen too.

My rating 4 **** out of 5 *****

3. The Breville 800JEXL Juice Fountain Elite 1000-Watt Juice Extractor Cost price approx. $299.00

Available on Amazon.com.

Product Features

- 1000-watt juicer with two speeds for soft and hard veggies and fruits, high (13,000 RPM) and low (6,500 RPM)

- 3" feeding tube no cutting of fruit or vegetables needed.

- Die-cast steel housing; stainless-steel micromesh filter; titanium-plated cutting disk

- Circular 3-inch feed tube accommodates whole fruits and vegetables

Product description

The Height of juice feeding tap is positioned for large glasses. Dish washer-safe parts. The Breville 800JEXL Juice Fountain Elite with 1000 watts is described by the maker as super-efficient.

It boosts an Italian made electronic motor that increases power while juicing to maintain its filter revolutions. It has TWO variable speeds for soft and hard fruits and has a 3" feed tube that minimizes cutting and preparation and feeding time.

Overall a beautiful stainless die cast steel design, a stylish fitting accessory makes it a work of art on the for every kitchen countertop.

MY REVIEW

This is one of the best. It has a high juice yield (produces really dry pulp), it can juice grasses and greens efficiently (wheatgrass, parsley, spinach etc.), and low temperatures and rpm minimize oxidation so live juices lasts a longer. The most attractive claims for this juicer were the fast juicing speed, relatively easy cleanup, and the wide mouth (3" round) opening.

My rating 5 ***** out of 5 *****

CHAPTER 6

WHAT ARE THE HEALTH BENEFITS OF EACH FRUIT VEGETABLE AND HERB USED IN THE GREEN JUICE DETOX DIET?

AVOCADO

Have 35% more potassium than bananas. They are rich in vitamin B, E and K. have high fibre content help lower blood cholesterol levels.

APPLES

Good for liver and intestines, relieves diarrhea.

BLACKBERRIES

Prevent diarrhea, help eliminate phlegm.

BLUEBERRIES

Help to strengthen your immune system, can lower your fever.

CHERRIES

Strengthen blood, very good for colon and menstrual problems.

GRAPES

Purify and strengthen blood, good for colon.

LEMONS

GOOD FOR LIVER AND GALLBLADDER, HELPS WITH ALLERGIES, ASTHMA, CARDIOVASCULAR DISEASE, AND COLDS.

ORANGES

Strengthens your immune and nervous system, good for cardiovascular disease, obesity, and varicose veins.

PEACHES

Improve your skin health, help detoxify.

PEARS

Help to lower blood pressure, good for gallbladder.

PINEAPPLE

Good for eyes and skin, helps with allergies, arthritis, inflammation and edema.

STRAWBERRIES

Cleansing to the blood, strengthen nerves.

WATERMELON

Good for kidneys, helps with edema.

What are the health benefits of Vegetable Juices?

Beetroot

This is good for your blood, liver and can help with arthritis and menstrual problems.

Cabbage

Eases your colon, helps with ulcers and colitis.

Carrot

Numerous benefits for eyes and skin, fights infection, helps with arthritis and osteoporosis.

Celery

A strong detoxifier, really healthy for your kidneys.

Cucumber

Helpful towards dealing with edema and diabetes.

Dandelion

This is a great detoxifier.

Leafy Greens

A purifier, good for your skin, digestive problems and obesity.

Onion

Helps lower blood pressure and aides your colon.

Potatoes

These are good for your intestines and also counteracts excess acidity in your stomach.

RADISH
Good for liver.

SPINACH
Blood builder, helps treat eczema.

TOMATOES
Help your digestive system.

WHEATGRASS
Good for blood, liver, intestines and your breath.

ZUCCHINI

Zucchinis are an extremely rich source of foliates, potassium, and vitamin A. You can also get a good portion of magnesium and manganese from your serving of zucchini.

Health benefits of raw zucchini are the enhanced absorption of vital nutrients present in the fruit.

When consumed in raw form, ensure that the zucchini is not too mature or too long as it can be fibrous. Zucchini is best consumed in the form of its juice and also steamed for soups as well.

The health benefits of zucchini juice can be felt in the form of a total body cleansing. With its high water content zucchini juice is highly satisfying and treats your body with excellent nourishments of vitamin A and C and these other vital minerals.

Zucchini gives you a plentiful supply of vitamin A, C, E, and K and an incredible source of calcium for body, to repair and heal from sudden sugar attacks on the body.

Also magnesium, zinc, manganese, calcium, potassium and copper are found in zucchini.

WHAT ARE THE HEALTH BENEFITS OF JUICED HERBS?

GARLIC

Garlic Lowers your blood pressure, fights germs, good for allergies, colds, cardiovascular disease, and diabetes.

HORSERADISH

Acts as a disinfectant and a diuretic, diuretics are used to treat heart failure liver cirrhosis hypertension and certain kidney disease.

Some diuretics, such as acetazolamide helps to make the urine more alkaline free and are helpful in increasing excretion of substances in the cases of overdose or poisoning.

PARSLEY

A sprig of parsley can provide much more than a decoration on your plate. Parsley contains two types of unusual components that provide unique health benefits.

The first type is volatile oil components, the second type is flavonoids.

Parsley's volatile oils myristicin have been shown to inhibit tumour formation in animal studies, and particularly, tumour formation in the lungs.

The flavonoids in parsley especially luteolin have been shown to function as antioxidants that combine with highly reactive oxygen-containing molecules (called oxygen radicals) and help prevent oxygen-based damage to cells.

Parsley is also an excellent source of two vital nutrients Vitamin C and Vitamin A (notably through its concentration of the pro-vitamin A carotenoid, beta-carotene).

Beta-carotene, another important antioxidant, works in the fat-soluble areas of the body. Diets with beta-carotene-rich foods are also associated with a reduced risk for the development and progression of conditions like atherosclerosis, diabetes, and colon cancer.

Like vitamin C, beta-carotene may also be helpful in reducing the severity of asthma, osteoarthritis, and rheumatoid arthritis. Beta-carotene is converted by the body to vitamin A. Vitamin A a nutrient that's is so important to a strong immune system that its nickname is the "anti-infective vitamin."

Parsley is a good source of folic acid, one of the most important B vitamins. While it plays numerous roles in the body, one of its most critical roles in relation to cardiovascular health is its necessary participation in the process through which the body converts homocysteine into benign molecules.

Homocysteine is a potentially dangerous molecule that, at high levels, can directly damage blood vessels. High levels are associated with a significantly increased risk of heart attack and stroke in people with atherosclerosis or diabetic heart disease.

Enjoying foods rich in folic acid, like parsley, is an exceptionally good idea for individuals who either have, or wish to prevent, these diseases.

Folic acid is also a critical nutrient for proper cell division and is therefore vitally important for cancer-prevention in two areas of the body that contain rapidly dividing cells—the colon, and in women, the cervix.

The findings, presented in the Annals of the Rheumatic Diseases were drawn from a study of more than 20,000 subjects who kept diet diaries and were arthritis-free when the study began.

Subjects who consumed the lowest amounts of vitamin C-rich foods were more than three times more likely to develop arthritis than those who consumed the highest amounts.

So… next time parsley appears on your plate as a garnish, recognize its true worth and its abilities to improve your health. Also as an added bonus, you'll enjoy parsley's amazing ability to cleanse your palate and your breath at the end of your meal.

WATERCRESS

Detoxifier, good for anaemia and colds.

CAYENNE PEPPER

One of the most powerful herbs in the world with health properties including anti irritant, anti-cold or flu agent and anti-fungal properties.

It also helps with migraines, anti-allergen, aids digestion, prevents and treats blood clots, helps sweat during detox ridding the body of toxins and many other health benefits including a possible anti-cancer agent.

Cayenne pepper supports weight loss, lowers appetite, improves heart and blood pressure, helps with gum disease, and is a topical remedy… Just to name a few.

CORDYCEPS

This is very controversial, this mushroom is believed by both traditional herbalists and many Western scientists, to be one of the most potent and health improving herbs in the world.

Modern science however has very little knowledge about it.

The majority of facts and results have been taken from the studies done by Scientists in China.

It belongs to the family of mushrooms, fungus. The fruiting body of Cordyceps looks like grass. Among the numerous species, Cordyceps sinensis is the most famous due to its curing properties.

The Chinese discovered its powers many centuries ago, having observed that sheep that grazed on Cordyceps were stronger and healthier.

Traditional herbalists began using the fungus for curing many diseases in humans. Cordyceps was believed to be a cure-all herb, able to fortify all the body's systems, providing anti-aging, immune boosting, and strength increasing affects.

SALVIA ROOT

Salvia Root is a traditional Chinese herb that has increasingly become important in the West for supporting cardiovascular health and improving your liver function.

It helps to revitalize and detoxify the blood and it is one of the most highly regarded circulatory tonics. Salvia Root has been shown to inhibit bacterial growth, reduce fevers, diminishes inflammation, ease's skin problems and aids urinary excretion of toxins.

Salvia Root is a member of the multi-species Salvia genus family, and despite the fact that any herb of this genus may be called sage there are significant differences in medicinal components in the tops and roots that influence their uses.

GINGER ROOT

Ginger or ginger root is consumed as a delicacy, medicine or a spice. Preliminary research indicates that there is nine compounds found in ginger that may bind to your serotonin receptors.

This may influence gastrointestinal function and promotes the production of bile.

Ginger is well known as a remedy for nausea, travel sickness, and indigestion, colic, irritable bowel, loss of appetite, chills, colds, flu, poor circulation, menstrual cramps, dyspepsia (bloating, heartburn, flatulence), indigestion and gastrointestinal problems.

Ginger is a powerful anti-inflammatory herb and there has been much recent interest in its use for joint problems. It has also been recognised for arthritis, fevers, headaches, toothaches, coughs, bronchitis, osteoarthritis, rheumatoid arthritis, to ease tendonitis, lower cholesterol and blood-pressure and aid in preventing internal blood clots.

Ginger oil has been shown to prevent skin cancer in mice and a study at the University of Michigan demonstrated that gingerols could kill ovarian cancer cells.

CHAPTER 7

DAY 1.

HOW TO START THE 1-3 DAY GREEN JUICING DETOX DIET.

The night before starting your 1-3 day juicing detox diet it is advised that you take a laxative herbal tea.

The first morning and each morning following you should take a lukewarm glass of purified filtered water with one teaspoon of uniodized sea salt. The salt water is absorbed quickly in to your bloodstream and helps to flush out the toxins in your digestive tract.

The herbal tea also helps alongside the salt water to rid the waste from the body OR alternatively a lemon juice detox-diet recipe can replace this after the first day.

Between the saltwater mixture and the nightly herbal laxative tea you are to consume 4-6 glasses of the juicing detox-diet meal full of anti-oxidants fibre and protein per day.

Please note due to the potent nature of the live juices you are recommended to dilute this by at least a quarter, of which is 1 part water (purified filtered) to 3 parts juice.

No solid foods may be consumed but you can drink as much purified filtered water alongside the juicing mixture as you want. You may also occasionally drink green tea or peppermint tea with no sugar added as your daily treat.

It is advised that the juicing mixture is made up in larger containers that helps bulk servings and prevents you from tiring of individual servings.

However, this is optional and by extracting the juice from a fruit or vegetable, you are taking in the valuable enzymes, nutrients, vitamins and minerals without your body having all the work of breaking down the fibres.

Also bear in mind the benefit of the live nutrients released by juicing deteriorates over a short period of time (15-20) minutes. Using a vacuum-sealed drinks container allows you to store the juice for approximately 12 hours in the fridge without loss of the live nutrients.

An important part of your detox is to rest, drink 2-4 glasses of purified filtered water daily and take a low to moderate rate of exercise like walking the dog, fast walking or a low intensity exercise class.

Its 1-3 days so know your limits…

A TYPICAL DAY OF THE DETOX DIET.

4-6 Detox Juice Drinks per day.
2-4 Purified Filtered Water.

FIRST THING

Flush saltwater mixture or 1 Cleanse lemon juice, 1 drink of purified filtered water.

BREAKFAST

1 drink purified filtered water. 1 nutritional energy juice drink to get you started. Try the Vegetable Super Juice. This juice gives your energy levels a boost, awakens your digestive system whilst giving your body nutrition.

If you are keen to get your '5-a-Day' this is an excellent start for your detox!

LUNCH

1 drink purified filtered water. Look at 2 nutritional recipes and target different areas of your body, i.e. if your immune system is low, you suffer from digestion problems or you have high cholesterol then choose the recipe that benefits you.

DINNER

Drink 1-2 purified filtered water. Look at 2 specific areas depending on what you want from your detox whilst balancing out the nutrients.

A great one can be the soup recipe that includes the broccoli soup or the Green Juice (Green Lemonade) detox diet juice recipe. This one is a great recipe that you can drink every day, tastes great and makes you feel amazing!

Once you're at the end of your first detox diet here are some suggestions you can adopt into your everyday life and diet:-

* Drink at least one detox juice a day, this can be a cleansing juice or energy breakfast juice drink.

* Lightly steam all your vegetables allowing it to lock in all the nutrients and great taste.

* Reduce or cut out refined sugars, also paying attention to the sugars contained in foods.

* Increase the consumption of organic foods where you can, if you have space, why not set up a raised garden and grow a lot of your own vegetables? At least you know where your produce is coming from and you know it's truly organic.

* Use herbs on your everyday foods like the amazing cayenne pepper, sprinkled over white / red meats or fish, you can also add cordyceps, parsley, ginger root and salvia root to your foods and juicing drinks too.

* Keep your body hydrated, drink purified filtered water. Did you know about 80% of people are dehydrated? Your body can't

determine hunger between thirst and you generally turn to food when in fact you just need re hydrated.

* Every three months whilst maintaining the healthy detox diet, complete the detox cleanse diet for your whole body.

JUICING DIET RECIPE'S (1 SERVING)

JUICING DETOX-DIET – CARROT JUICE
5 large carrots

Carrots are beneficial for helping regenerate the mucous membranes of the colon wall. This is due to their generous supply of vitamin A, which is needed for the health of all mucous membranes in the body. Carrot juice is also great for bulking up the faeces.

JUICING DETOX-DIET – APPLE AND PEAR
2 Apples

2 Pears

No need to peel the apples and pears, this will add some fibre to the juice. Apple and pear juices are great for helping the bowels move, so this is also a great constipation remedy.

JUICING DETOX-DIET – LEMON JUICE
2 lemons

Add water to dilute

Only juice the flesh of the lemons. Add water to your taste. This is a great juice to take on an empty stomach before breakfast. It has a great flushing affect, and is actually very beneficial for the kidneys and liver. If you warm it up a little it can help move the bowels even more, but don't overdo the heat. Remember the hotter the juice, the more the nutrients are destroyed.

JUICING DETOX-DIET – ACL COLON CLEANSE

4 Carrots

1 Apple

1 Lemon

By extracting the juice from a fruit or vegetable, you are taking in the valuable enzymes, nutrients, vitamins and minerals without all the work of having your body break down the fibres.

VEGETABLE SUPER JUICE (SERVES 1)

1/2 Cucumber

2 Sticks of celery

1-2 Handfuls of spinach

½ Zucchini

4 Lettuce leaves

Other greens as desired.

This juice is a popular one for your breakfast as it gives your energy levels a boost, wakens your digestive system whilst giving your body nutrition, yet giving you a gentle start to the day. If you are keen to get '5-a-Day' this is an excellent start!

Juice all ingredients and mix 50/50 with purified filtered water. Add lemon juice to taste.

Optional boosters: Parsley and fresh alfalfa sprouts

HEALING DETOX JUICE (SERVES 1)

1 1/2 - 2 Carrots

60g Fresh Spinach

Handful of Flat Leaf Parsley

1 – 1 1/2 Sticks of Celery

A sweeter more subtle juice that is full of nutrition. The combination of the carrots, spinach and parsley provide an excellent source of antioxidants, while the celery helps us with its cleansing properties.

Juice all ingredients but remember you should put the celery through last then mix with water to taste or you can drink it neat.

CHAPTER 8

*H*OW TO FINISH THE GREEN JUICING DETOX DIET.

Before finishing the juicing diet you should know you <u>should not</u> start eating solids straight away. Coming off the diet is one of the most important parts to the juicing diet-detox and should be done properly.

DAY 4.

Have a few pieces of fruit, lightly steamed vegetables for the 4th day along with 1–3 glasses of juicing detox drink, and as much purified filtered water as you need.

DAY 5.

You can start to eat brown rice, beans, eggs, whole wheat bread and salad with 1-2 glasses of juicing detox drink.

DAY 6.

It is recommended that you have meat, white meat or fish is recommended and introduce your main diet foods.

After your detox you should be consuming some of the fruit and vegetables you have used in your 3-day Amazing Juicing detox-diet.

Also try adding Cayenne pepper and other herbs to your meals, like meats, fish etc. The health benefits are truly AMAZING.

CONGRATULATIONS AND WELL DONE...

At this point you will have successfully completed the Green Juice detox-diet and will feel the benefits discussed throughout this book. I sincerely hope you enjoyed this book and are able to make some of exciting recipes and even develop some of your own. See Chapter 9 &10.

Oliver Michaels

Chapter 9

Amazing 'easy to Make Juicing Detox Diet Recipes.

The success of this juicing detox-diet plan is based on improving the liver function through your simple 'easy make' recipe dietary habits which will allow you to achieve many of the health benefits, especially your weight control and internal cleansing of your body.

People who have struggled for years with excessive weight or health problems have found that their liver was the missing link to achieving good health.

Please Note:

During the juicing detox-diet try to limit fruits with excess sugars, like pineapple. It is advised not to use too many high sugar ingredients in your detox drinks.

The sugar will coat what the drink has just cleaned, thus defeating the whole process.

you're looking for a recipe ingredient to add taste to your juice then try adding Apple, ginger or Carrot.

Carrot, Cucumber & Lime Detox Juicer Recipe.

3 Carrots

1/2 Large cucumber

1/2 Lime

Juice all ingredients and enjoy this refreshing delicious juice.

CELERY, CARROT & PARSLEY DETOX DIET JUICE RECIPE.

3 Celery sticks

3 Carrots

1 Bunch parsley

Process the ingredients above through your juicer. This is an amazing detoxifier and will really boost your immunity too!

TOMATO, LETTUCE & CUCUMBER DETOX DIET JUICE RECIPE.

3 Large, ripe tomatoes

6 Leaves leafy lettuce (I prefer romaine or kale)

Cucumber (about a 2-inch piece)

1 Garlic clove (optional)

Handful of fresh cilantro or parsley

Small wedge of lemon or lime

Juice all the ingredients.

CARROT RADISH APPLE BEET LEMON AMAZING DETOX DIET JUICE RECIPE.

1 Large carrot

10 Radishes

1 Apple

1 Beetroot

Then juice and add finely grated zest of 2 lemons

1/4 cups naturally sparkling mineral water (optional)

Juice the first 4 ingredients. Add the lemon juice and zest. If you want a longer fizzy drink, add the mineral water.

Vitamin A is the essential vitamin for healthy, radiant skin. You'll get it in abundance from the carrots in this juicing recipe.

The additional bonus comes from the radishes, their natural constituents stimulates the cleansing function of your liver.

This is the perfect juicing detox recipe when you've been a bit overindulged or your digestive system seems to be slightly sluggish.

APPLE CELERY SWISS CHARD KALE DETOX DIET JUICE RECIPE.

1 Big handful of kale or Swiss chard

2 Celery stalks

2 Apples

Process in your juicer and enjoy this delicious recipe.

Carrot, Cabbage & Romaine detox diet Juice Recipe.

6 Leaves romaine lettuce

2 Leaves green cabbage

2 Carrots

Juice the veggies and enjoy your detox.

Fresh Greens and Oranges detox diet Juice Recipe.

6 leaves green leafy lettuce or kale or a big handful of spinach

2 oranges

Process these through your juicer.

This is a very tasty juicing detox recipe. Enjoy!

Tomato, Carrot, Celery & Lemon detox diet Juice Recipe.

3 Ribs of celery

2 Tomatoes

2 Carrots

A squeeze of lemon juice

Process all but the lemon juice through your juicer and then add the squeeze of a fresh lemon, stir well before you drink! Enjoy!

BEETROOT, GRAPEFRUIT & CELERY DETOX DIET JUICE RECIPE.

2 Beetroots

1 Grapefruit

2 Celery sticks

This one is an earthy detox juice that soothes your whole body.

You will not only get great detox qualities from this juice, you will also be re-energized, and this will also boost your immune system and beautify your skin.

APPLE & BEETROOT DETOX DIET JUICE RECIPE.

3 Apples

1/2 Beetroot

This juice will be deep red in colour. It tastes earthy but the apples make it quite sweet and very tasty. This juice has many detox properties – your body will love it!

CARROT, APPLE & ZUCCHINI DETOX DIET JUICE RECIPE.

3 large Carrots

2 Apples unpeeled

2 Medium Zucchini unpeeled

This juice will give you a burst of energy after just one glass. The juice tastes incredible too, it has many amazing detox properties!

CELERY, PEAR & WATERCRESS DETOX DIET JUICE RECIPE.

3 Whole celery sticks

2 Medium pears

1 Bunch of watercress

Process the two pears, celery and watercress all together through your juicer.

This is a beautiful green juice that is great for detoxing your body. As well as boosting your immune system this juicing recipe also improves your digestion.

SPINACH, APPLE & CARROT DETOX DIET JUICE RECIPE.

1 Handful of spinach

1 Large Apple

5 Carrots

Process the ingredients through your juicer.

This is a great detox juicer recipe that will improve your stomach and digestive system.

GINGER, CARROT & APPLE DETOX DIET JUICE RECIPE.

1 Medium apple

8 Carrots

1/4 to 1/2 inch Ginger root (to your personal taste)

Push the ginger through your juicer hopper along with the carrots and apple whole this is a great cleansing juicing detox and also tastes great too!

PINEAPPLE, CELERY, GINGER & FLAXSEED DETOX DIET JUICE RECIPE.

2 Cups of pineapple

3 Celery sticks

1 Inch ginger root

1/8 Teaspoon flaxseed oil

Process the celery, pineapple and the ginger root through your juicer. Pour contents into a glass. Then add the flaxseed oil and mix thoroughly.

You may want to make this juice and then put in a container cup that has a lid - add the juice and the flaxseed oil - shake to mix. Pour contents into a glass and enjoy!

This juicing detox recipe is a tasty detox and has a very beneficial combination of minerals, antioxidants and healthy fats.

Great for your promotion of healthy joints and it reduces any of your body's inflammations.

APPLE, RASPBERRY, ORANGE & SPIRULINA DETOX DIET JUICE RECIPE.

2 Apples

2 Cups of raspberries

1 Orange

1 Teaspoon Spirulina (This is optional)

Juice the apples, raspberries and orange.

If you add the spirulina you need to pour the juice into a container cup that has a lid.

Add the Spirulina and then close the lid – shake well to mix. Then drink and Enjoy!

GREEN JUICE (GREEN LEMONADE) DETOX DIET JUICE RECIPE.

1 Head of romaine lettuce

5 to 6 Stalks of kale

2 Sweet apples (Use Fuji or Pink Lady apples)

1 Whole lemon (organic is best so you don't have to peel it)

1 to 2 Tablespoons fresh ginger root (optional)

Process the vegetables and fruit through your juicer.

This recipe will give you approximately 2 large glasses of juice – remember you can half the ingredients or put the 2nd glass in your fridge and drink it throughout the day.

This is a great recipe that you can drink every day. It has great taste and makes you feel amazing!

APPLE, TOMATO AND BERRY DETOX DIET JUICE RECIPE.

2 Large apples (Fiji or Pink Lady)

1 Large tomato

1/3 Cup raspberries

Juice the apple, tomato and raspberries into a glass. Stir juice and drink.

APPLE, CELERY AND SPINACH DETOX DIET JUICE RECIPE.

2 Large apples (Fiji or Pink Lady)

2 Large stalks celery

1/2 Cup packed spinach leaves

1/4 Teaspoon cayenne pepper

Juice apples, celery and spinach into a glass. Stir pepper into juice and drink.

TOMATO, CARROT, CUCUMBER AND LEMON DETOX DIET JUICE RECIPE.

3 Large tomatoes

3 Large carrots

1 Medium cucumber

1/2 A small lemon

APPLE, SPINACH AND MINT DETOX DIET JUICE RECIPE.

2 medium apples (Fiji or pink lady)

1 Cup of spinach leaves

2 Large carrots

1 Medium stalk of celery

1 Medium cucumber

2 Tablespoon packed mint

Juice apple, spinach, carrot, celery, cucumber and mint into a glass. Stir juice and drink.

APPLE, PARSLEY, CARROT AND BEETROOT DETOX DIET JUICE RECIPE.

2 Medium apples (Fiji or Pink Lady)

3 Tablespoons packed parsley

3 Large carrots

1 Beetroot

Juice apples, parsley, carrots and beetroot into a glass. Stir juice and drink.

TOMATO, CARROT, CUCUMBER AND LEMON DETOX DIET JUICE RECIPE.

3 Large tomatoes

3 Large carrots

1 Medium cucumber

1/2 A small lemon

Juice tomato, carrot, cucumber and lemon into a glass. Stir juice and drink.

CARROT, CUCUMBER AND TOMATO DETOX DIET JUICE RECIPE.

5 Large carrots

1 Small cucumber

1 Small tomato

1 Small stalk celery

1/2 Cup romaine lettuce

3 Tablespoons parsley

Juice carrot, cucumber, tomato, celery, lettuce and parsley into a large glass. Stir juice and drink. This juice is great for your colon and would really help you jump start a colon cleanse.

Continue the above for up to 3 days.

Juicing of fresh fruits and vegetables in a juicer detox process can be one of the most beneficial steps you can take to provide good nourishing fuel for your body.

Remember you should mix up your recipes to vary the taste and effect that the recipe has on your body, you can utilise the *create your own ingredients plan* in chapter 10 to make your own amazing recipes too..!

CHAPTER 10

BONUS RECIPES...

WARM / WINTER SOUP JUICING DETOX-DIET RECIPES.

HIGHLY ENERGISING SOUP
Serves 2

This is definitely a highly energising soup and is a big favourite while on a detox diet. Contains avocado that is high in EFAs and cucumber that is well known for its cleansing properties. The taste of this soup can be dramatically altered by the use of the herbs and spices mentioned or by alternating between the lemon and lime.

1 Avocado

2 Spring onions

1/2 Red or green pepper

1 Cucumber

2 Handfuls of spinach

1/2 clove of garlic

100ml of light vegetable Bouillon (yeast free)

Juice of 1 lemon or lime

Optional: coriander, parsley, and cumin.

Blend the avocado and stock to form a light paste and then add the other ingredients and BLEND.

WARM BROCCOLI SOUP
Serves 2

This is definitely a winter favourite and destroys the myth that all raw food has to be cold and unwelcoming! By steaming the broccoli for just 5-6 minutes, the meal remains raw, but gains enough warmth to give that filling comforting feeling of soup. The texture given by the broccoli and the kick of the ginger makes this an excellent choice.

1/2 Avocado

6 -8 decent size broccoli heads

1/3 Red Onion

1 Celery Stick

½ Zucchini

Big Handful of Spinach

An Inch of Root Ginger

Cumin (Optional)

Lightly steam the broccoli (5-6 minutes) and put with all ingredients in a blender. Add garlic, pepper, and real salt to taste. The heat from the broccoli makes this a lovely, gently warmed soup great for winter.

Autumn Tomato & Avocado Soup

Serves 2

This is a nice soup to have either cold (a bit like gazpacho) or warmed (on a slightly chilly morning or evening)

5 Large ripe (preferably vine) tomatoes.

1 Ripe avocado

1 Spring onion

1/4 Cup ground almonds (freshly done yourself, not packet)

1-cup broth from Swiss Vegetable Bouillon

1/4 Teaspoon dill seed

Dash cayenne pepper

Add sea salt & cracked black pepper to taste.

All you need to do is place all of the ingredients into a blender (except one of the tomatoes) and blend! Depending on whether you are going cold or warm - then place the soup into a pan and warm very slightly. Warming but don't boil or cook (not painful to put your finger into) still means that the soup is raw. Add the last tomato (sliced) on top and serve.

Conclusion

Detox dieting is beneficial even if you're a health "addict", to complete a periodical cleanse will help you kick start your body into losing weight, clear up bloated or digestion issues and will boost your immune system too.

You should ideally complete the 3-day juicing detox diet once every 1 - 3 months and have introduced a lot of the detox diet into your everyday life. I suggest completing your detox at the beginning of every season (spring, summer autumn, winter).

By doing this regular detox I prevent my overall diet from straying back into unhealthy eating. Remember eating is largely social and habitual, we are seduced and bombarded with social engagements, adverts, smells and experiences of everyday foods which can put us back into the realm of unhealthy eating.

I would NEVER recommend doing anything more than a 3-day detox diet more than once every month. If you're feeling you need to detox your body and cleanse more often than that, your diet needs fixing…fast!!

During this book you have learnt to incorporate foods into your daily diet, facilitate your body's own detox and remove the foods that inhibit your body's natural detox.

Oliver Michaels.

CONTACT ME

Well we're nearly at the end of my book, so tell me what did you think? Did I really help you? How can I improve and get better? I am currently writing my new book The Ultimate Juicing Bible, *(subscribe here and you will get this copy free when it's released mid 2013 along with any other new book I release)* it will have even more juicing and diet information and more amazing recipes too. What would you like to see from this book?

Please email me and let me know… I do hope you agreed that there were some amazing recipes, juicing information and all you need to start juicing in this book.

Also if you feel you have any questions for me…**Please, please, please email me at** olivermichaels.author@hotmail.com.

I personally read and answer every email.

MY APPEAL TO YOU

I am continuously researching and improving my books, I want to provide you with the latest and best information for your juicing diet and healthy lifestyle.

If you found this book helpful **I would very, very, very much appreciate** a quick review from you. You see, I want to over-deliver the quality of information in my book at a truly amazing price.

A 4 or 5 star review is really and truly like leaving me a $25 tip. I read every single review and beam with pride knowing someone enjoyed my book and more importantly they have introduced juicing into their daily lives.

I only want honest reviews from beautiful (or handsome) readers who do really like my book….☺

If you have any questions, ideas suggestions or criticisms for me then also…**Please please email me at** :-
olivermichaels.author@hotmail.com THANK YOU.

Oliver Michaels

Scan this QR code with your smart phone to order additional copies of this book.

Createspace edition original © 2012.

Glossary.

Amino acids

Amino acids are the building blocks of the proteins that are found in our bodies. The human body can produce 10 of its 20 amino acids, but the other 10, which are called essential amino acids can only be obtained by eating the right foods.

Beta-carotene

Beta-carotene is one of a group of natural chemicals known as carotene or carotenoids. Carotenes are responsible for the orange colour of many fruits and vegetables such as carrots, pumpkins, and sweet potatoes. Beta-carotene is converted in the body to vitamin A. It is an antioxidant, like vitamins E and C

Cholecystokinin

Cholecystokinin is a peptide hormone of the gastrointestinal system that is responsible for stimulating the digestion of fat and protein. Cholecystokinin was previously called pancreozymin, and is synthesised by I-cells in the small intestine and secreted in the duodenum, the first segment of the small intestine. It causes the release of digestive enzymes and bile from the pancreas and gallbladder, respectively. It also acts as a hunger suppressant.

Cleanse

A body cleanse instantly improves your health. A body detox aids with allergies, fatigue and chronic health problems.

DETOX

Detox may refer to: Detoxification, the process, real or perceived of removing toxins from the body.

DIET

Your diet is quite simply, what you eat. There are two aspects to your diet: what foods you eat and how much of them you eat.

GLUTATHIONE

Glutathione is a small protein composed of three amino acids-cysteine, glutamic acid and glycine it's an amazing anti-oxidant. It is produced in the human liver and plays a key role in intermediary metabolism, immune response and health and Glutathione. This protein reduces the outward signs of aging such as age spots and wrinkles. People suffering from immune-suppression, stress and lack of sleep or any chronic illness may need more glutathione.

L-CYSTEINE

L-cysteine is a naturally occurring amino acid that is classified as a protein amino acid. One of the main functions of L-cysteine is the promotion of stomach lining health and also the correction of situations where the absorption of essential nutrients from food sources takes place.

L-GLUTAMINE

L-glutamine also known as glutamine is a non-essential amino acid. This means that it does not need to be obtained from dietary sources, since the human body can make it on its own. L-glutamine is the most abundant amino acid in the human body and is also found in a wide variety of foods. It is also used in dietary supplements and is claimed to be useful for a variety of different conditions, such as depression anxiety and insomnia, and various nutritional disorders.

MICRO NUTRIENTS

Micronutrients, as opposed to macronutrients (protein, carbohydrates and fat), are comprised of vitamins and minerals that are required in small quantities to ensure normal metabolism, growth and physical well-being.

MINERALS

Minerals these are inorganic nutrients that also play a key role in ensuring health and well-being. They include the trace elements copper, iodine, iron, manganese, selenium and zinc together with the macro elements calcium, magnesium, potassium and sodium. As with vitamins, minerals are found in small quantities within the body and they are obtained from a wide variety of foods.

NAC AMINO ACID

NAC was first developed as a therapeutic for its ability to break up mucus in the lungs in conditions like bronchitis. However, research into NAC's other amazing benefits soon gained momentum. This was largely due to NAC's ability to raise glutathione levels in the body, which is significant because glutathione is one of our body's most important antioxidants. In recent years it has become apparent that NAC has great potential not only for raising your body's antioxidant levels, but also for preventing heart disease, memory loss, cancer, and even aging itself. It is an ingredient used in medication and often used by hospitals, can be found in Tylenol.

PHOSPHOLIPIDS

Phospholipids are a class of lipids that are a major component of all cell membranes as they can form lipid bilayers.

PHYTONUTRIENTS

Phytonutrients are nutrients derived from plant material that have been shown to be necessary for sustaining human life. Phytochemicals are non-nutritive plant chemicals that contain protective disease-preventing compounds.

PURIFIED WATER

Purified water is water from any source that is physically processed to remove impurities. Distilled water and deionized (DI) water are the most common forms of purified water, but water can also be purified by other processes including reverse osmosis, carbon filtration, microfiltration and so on.

TOXINS

Toxins, derived from the Ancient Greeks. Toxins are a poisonous substance produced within living cells or organisms, synthetic substances created by artificial processes are therefore excluded. The term was first used by organic chemist Ludwig Brieger (1849–1919). For a toxic substance not produced within living organisms, the terms "toxicant" and "toxics" are also sometimes used.

Medical Disclaimer.

THIS BOOK IS NOT DESIGNED TO, AND DOES NOT, PROVIDE MEDICAL ADVICE. ALL CONTENT ("CONTENT"), INCLUDING TEXT, GRAPHICS, IMAGES AND INFORMATION AVAILABLE ON OR THROUGHOUT THIS BOOK ARE FOR GENERAL INFORMATIONAL PURPOSES ONLY GAINED THROUGH THE AUTHORS EXTENSIVE RESEARCH AND EXPERIENCES.

THE CONTENT IS NOT INTENDED TO BE A SUBSTITUTE FOR PROFESSIONAL MEDICAL ADVICE, DIAGNOSIS OR TREATMENT. NEVER DISREGARD PROFESSIONAL MEDICAL ADVICE, OR DELAY IN SEEKING IT, BECAUSE OF SOMETHING YOU HAVE READ IN THIS BOOK. NEVER RELY ON INFORMATION IN THIS BOOK IN PLACE OF SEEKING PROFESSIONAL MEDICAL ADVICE.

THE GREEN JUICE DETOX DIET AUTHOR IS NOT RESPONSIBLE OR LIABLE FOR ANY ADVICE, COURSE OF TREATMENT, DIAGNOSIS OR ANY OTHER INFORMATION, SERVICES OR PRODUCTS THAT YOU OBTAIN THROUGH THIS BOOK. YOU ARE ENCOURAGED TO CONFER WITH YOUR DOCTOR WITH REGARD TO INFORMATION CONTAINED IN OR THROUGH THIS BOOK. AFTER READING THE CONTENT FROM THIS BOOK, YOU ARE ENCOURAGED TO REVIEW THE INFORMATION CAREFULLY WITH YOUR PROFESSIONAL HEALTHCARE PROVIDER.

THE GREEN JUICE DETOX DIET © 2013.